AFTER ME, YOU COME FIRST

by

Sara Armstrong

and

Lillian Redding

ISBN 978-1-4357-0638-5

WE DEDICATE THIS BOOK

' To our foremothers who laid the foundation on which we are building our future.

' To the men in our lives, Carl, Bob, Tyler and Xavier, who give us support and motivated us to excel.

' To Alexis so that she may grow, prosper and blossom into the fullness of her womanhood.

' To all men and women so they may know their own worth and become their own best friend.

FOREWORD

Prisoners of Liberation

The five women gathered for a visit in the summer of 1848 had no idea the revolution they would begin. It was seventy years after the Revolutionary War where women had sacrificed, struggled and died along side men in the fight for American independence. But life did not change much for women after the war. They did not enjoy even minimal rights of citizenship.

Elizabeth Cady Stanton was the spark that lit the fire of the women's movement. Her conversation with four friends over tea that afternoon was the basis for the world's first Women's Rights Convention held in at Wesleyan Chapel in Seneca Falls, New York, July 19 -20, 1848. It was described as "A convention to discuss the social, civil, and religious condition and rights of women." The women used the Declaration of Independence as a template for writing a Declaration of Sentiments. Some of the

grievances listed were:

- Married women were legally dead in the eyes of the law
- Women were not allowed to vote
- Women had to submit to laws when they had no voice in their formation
- Married women had no property rights
- Husbands had legal power over and responsibility for their wives to the extent that they could imprison or beat them with impunity
- Divorce and child custody laws favored men, giving no rights to women
- Women had to pay property taxes although they had no representation in the levying of these taxes
- Most occupations were closed to women and when women did work they were paid only a fraction of what men earned
- Women were not allowed to enter professions such as medicine or law
- Women had no means to gain an education since no college or university would accept women students
- With only a few exceptions, women were not allowed to participate in the affairs of the church
- Women were robbed of their self-confidence and self-respect, and were made totally dependent on men

Elizabeth Cady Stanton wrote: "The women of this country

ought be enlightened in regard to the laws under which they

live, that they may no longer publish their degradation by

declaring themselves satisfied with their present position,

nor their ignorance, by asserting that they have all the

rights they want."

The flood gates of the women's movement were

opened and through them flowed Susan B Anthony,

Grandma Moses, Mary Kay Ash, Maria Callas, Charlotte

Bronte, Coco Chanel, Nikki Giovanni, Lillian Hellman,

Leontyne Price, Mae Jemison, Maya Angelou, Elizabeth

Blackwell, Oprah Winfrey, Sally Ride, Judith Jamison,

Lillian Carter, Ruth Westheimer, Bernice Johnson Reagon,

Katherine Hepburn, Rachel Carson, Margaret Mead, Betty

Freidan, Carole King, Shirley Chisolm, Margaret Thatcher,

Harriet Tubman, Dorothy Day, Bella Abzug, Barbara

Walters, Condolezza Rice, Judge Judy, Ellen Degeneres

and countless others who cut a pathway through the jungles

of limitation and discrimination.

Because of these fearless females, the 21st century

woman has more choices than ever, more freedom than

ever. But it doesn't necessarily make life easier. Women are still pulled and swayed by what they can do, what they want to do, what other people want, expect and approve of. We are buffeted by biology, economics, and the very human need for personal and spiritual fulfillment.

Early in our lives we learn that females play the major role in the reproductive process. We are given dolls to play with and told that one day when we are mothers we will do this or that. But even if we choose to follow our most basic biological urges, we find that is not as simple as it seems.

You are told that you are only allowed to have children under certain circumstances. You shouldn't be below a certain age because obviously you are incapable of raising a child and besides, what will people think. But you shouldn't be over a certain age, like 40, because obviously you are incapable of raising a child and besides what will people think.

Those women who want to have children but can't for whatever reason are allowed to adopt, use a surrogate or employ in vitro fertilization but only if they follow the rules about having a proper partner and being of proper age.

Should you choose not to have children and vigorously pursue a career, then obviously you are a coldhearted, calculating person who feels too inadequate to be a parent. You are filling up the hole in your maternal soul with money, drive and ambition. You are not feminine and are in fact trying to be a man or are struggling with your sexuality. You will live an empty miserable life and die old and alone in your penthouse and then what will people think.

If you do choose to have a career, find a job that is fulfilling and decide to stay in that job and not scratch and claw your way further up the corporate ladder, then obviously you just don't have what it takes to make in the working world and should have stayed home and had children.

And should you have the temerity to want both a family and a career, obviously you won't do either one properly. If you pursue your career to the highest, then your children will suffer irreparable damage because you were not at every single one of their soccer games, and didn't have milk and cookies ready everyday when they came home from school or never took your turn as snack mom at baseball practice. They will certainly be maladjusted, have ADHD, be incapable of maintaining a relationship and may possibly become raging sociopaths, which of course would all be your fault, and then what will people think. Also if you have a mate you must make sure that he/she does not feel threatened or inconvenienced by your desire to work. Because if they can't adjust, then the relationship may deteriorate and it will of course all be your fault, and what will people think.

If you arrange your work schedule to spend more time with your family then you are asking for special treatment. You want to have your career but are not willing to pay the price. If you ask you mate for help too often then you are a immature whiner and what will people think.

If you are a women (single, married, or divorced) who **must** work to support your family, then you obviously chose to marry someone who couldn't support you properly or you don't know how to manage your money or you need to go back to school and get a degree or get a better job and you probably shouldn't have had children in the first place. Your punishment for this is to devote yourself entirely to your children, not have a social life, not pursue you own dreams and be consumed with guilt throughout eternity.

All of your children must have college funds, trust funds and a car by age eighteen at the latest. If your kids have to work their way through school, get a job to support themselves, use public transportation or for whatever reason, don't go to college you really have some explaining to do. You must actively suffer from Empty Nest Syndrome and be willing to have the children move back in whenever they encounter even the slightest problem or bump on the road of life.

And if the twists and turns of life place you on public assistance or in a shelter or on the street, then you must really have done something wrong and you know what people will say, "How could you a 21st century woman end up like this with all the opportunities you have?"

Is the only way to be a successful homemaker mastering Martha Stewart's recipe for making marshmallows from scratch or knowing the perfect way to fold a fitted sheet? Are you a failure as a mother because there are times your children's behavior qualify you for a visit from Jojo the Supernanny? Does changing careers several times in a lifetime mean you are unfocused and flighty? Why is Brittany Spears repeatedly maligned for her parenting skills while NBA players suffer no consequences for fathering scores of children whom they never parent? Why are strippers vilified but men compete to be Chippendale dancers?

In spite of all the advances, women still are judged and evaluated differently than men. What is more important, women often judge each other more harshly than society does. We try and validate our choices by criticizing the choices of others. Of course not all women will agree on every subject. Discussion and debate are healthy but we must avoid at all costs becoming a house divided.

This book is intended to examine the major forces that impact the lives of women in this flat, small world. The primary message is that whatever path you choose or whichever journey is thrust upon you by genetics, circumstances or karma, the most important person in your life must be you. Being selfish is actually self-preservation because you won't be of any use to anyone if you misuse

yourself.

CHAPTER 1

Watching and Learning

Debates range in our society about gender identification and roles. Males are elected prom queens and women play football. The words traditional and non-traditional are becoming obsolete or at least being redefined.

How do we know what we are supposed to be as women? How do we learn how to act, what to aspire to, how to relate to the world? We learn by how we are treated by others and by watching others of our gender as we grow and mature. Increasingly we learn from portrayals in all types of media. All of these influences are folded into each woman's unique personality and genetic structure to make us what we are.

Our mothers, or mother figures are primary in their influence. We watch them as they go about their lives. We watch them handle relationships. We learn as they raise and discipline us and our siblings. We hear stories of their lives and their mothers' lives and it lays out a life road map for us.

Our father, or father figures are equally influential. We watch how they treat women and how those women react. We internalize how they treat us differently from our male counterparts. We learn what pleases them and what doesn't. We learn how to compete for them and to compete with them.

Maybe these influences are positive, loving and empowering. Maybe the example they set is negative, possibly abusive or degrading. If you grew up with an addicted parent, absent parent or violent parent it will show up in your life. Even if you commit yourself not to follow in their footsteps, that path is part of you and you must be aware of its influence. We aren't psychologists but from our own life experience, we know the power of these parental examples.

Lillian and I are profoundly influenced by my mother Sara Jones McWright. She was a strong willed, proud woman who operated on the principle that she was always right. She spoke with supreme confidence, did things her way and if you didn't agree with her it would be your own fault when you failed. She was also family oriented and of high moral and ethical character.

Sara McWright was one of the older girls in a family of twelve. She helped raise her younger siblings and as they left the nest, she stayed to take care of her aging parents, not marrying until she was 39 years old. She married Edward McWright a kind, mild-mannered man with a wonderful sense of humor. His mother died when he was six years old and he grew up with a distant, strict father. After a disastrous first marriage and bitter divorce he remained a bachelor of seventeen years before marrying again.

While Edward and Sara did talk and negotiate on matters of household finance etc., things were usually done Sara's way. Their only child, Sara Louise was their pride and joy. But they were determined that I wouldn't be spoiled. If there was only one apple left in the house, it would be split three ways. I had chores to do, was expected to work hard in school and was to be on my best behavior at all times.

Their daughter, Sara Louise, grew up smart, compliant, somewhat repressed and with some serious self-esteem issues. Her parents in their efforts to teach and protect her also smothered her. She lived at home while she went to college and when she graduated broke free and went half-way around the world to find herself. She joined the Peace Corps went to Uganda; married a Ugandan, had two children and lived through the madness of a dictator.

4

Since returning to the USA in 1977, I have been a single parent, a caregiver, a mayor and twice widowed. The basic skills I used to survive life's twists and turns were learned in my early years. [1]

Here is what Lillian has to say about what she learned from the women in her life:

Growing up I always had strong spirited women in my life as examples. I remember my African grandmother, Janet, as a very vocal and strong woman. We called her Ja-Ja which is grandmother in Lugisu, my father's native language.

It was obvious to anyone looking in from the outside that she was definitely the glue of the Wanambwa family. Whenever we would visit her in the village you could hear her out in the fields supervising the workers as they tended the crops. She could organize a meal in minutes or settle a family dispute with wisdom and humor.

---

[1] Go to www.sarmstrong.biz and read about the extraordinary life of Sara Armstrong , founder of Women of Authority and her riveting book *The Shattered Pearl.*

Ja-Ja was a woman of great faith who lived by the principles of her faith. She loved her children and grandchildren but never let their needs overcome her own. She helped when she believed it was appropriate and spoke the truth no matter how painful it might be.

My maternal grandmother helped raise me after my father died. We lived in little town Shorter, Alabama near her childhood home of Montgomery, Alabama. Sara Jones-McWright was truly the pillar of our family. She grew up taking care of her siblings and parents. She was a first grade teacher and that is something she never let you forget.

My grandmother always made sure that you learned a life lesson in everything you did. When we went to the store and the total was $ 8.51, she would give the cashier $10.00 and say to us, "How much change should I get?" My brother and I would have to come up with the right answer and check the change she received before we left the store.

She taught me to "act like a lady" and to behave as if "you had some home training." She insisted that we speak properly and above all to maintain our dignity no matter what the situation. She would say, "You are a valuable person. Never be anyone's doormat."

Now that I look back on my childhood I remember my grandmother cooking meals and working in the garden. She had her own way of doing household chores. Even though we had a dryer, we still had to hang the clothes outside on the clothesline so the sunshine could kill all the germs and give the clothes that fresh smell. We had to iron the bed sheets and t-shirts and jeans. You never left the house wrinkled or unkempt. I didn't know then that those chores were laying the ground work for the dedicated work ethic I possess today and I am thankful.

My mother and grandparents were very family oriented and instilled those values into us. On holidays we would pull out all the good china and silver and dress the table with fine linens, my grandfather would take us out into the woods to find a Christmas tree and cut it down to take home and we would string popcorn for the Christmas tree and decorate it together. My mother and grandmother would involve us in the holiday cooking and baking, allowing us to help make homemade rolls and cakes. We felt so proud and close when we did these things as a family. I try to share those types of events with my kids today, because when you get older those are the memories that never die and give you comfort.

My mother was widowed with two kids at a young age, and from the day the state trooper showed up at our house to tell us our Dad had been killed in a drunk driver accident the night before, my Mom was strong for all of us.

I remember at his funeral, I was only five yrs old and so confused, my Mom and I went to the bathroom in the funeral home before we went to the cemetery, and I saw one tear fall down her face, that she quickly wiped away. That is the only time I recall seeing her cry in my childhood. She was then taking care of me, my brother and both senior parents. She worked all the time, and then when she got home she had her kids wanting her full attention, my grandmother already had the grocery list written out and all the local stores mapped out, so she could use all her store coupons.

How did she do it? I never remember seeing her breakdown or screaming, yelling, etc. I never remember seeing her say "Hey I am taking a long bubble bath and pampering myself today." She always created special moments with us. Every summer we went on vacation and she drove the entire trip.

How did she hold it together in front of us? Did she have time to herself? My father died in 1978 when I was five, and I never saw my mother date anyone, until she met my stepfather when I was seventeen years old and in high school. Although I will be eternally grateful to my mother, seeing this superwoman in my eyes always giving, giving, and giving, I found that I also learned not to take care of myself. I was constantly concerned with the kids needs, my husbands needs, and always put my needs on the back burner.

I felt like it was a sign of weakness if I showed emotion, or was too tired to cook dinner every night. I truly had a perception that these women in my life never got weary, that they were never scared, that they never just wanted to stay in the bed and sleep. I often have tried to be that unachievable "Super Woman" but I now know that, they were tired, scared, and uncertain and did a great job of hiding it from their loved ones who depended on them and their strength.

One thing I have learned is that even though I do want my daughter to see that women are strong in many ways, and I want her to be confident in all that she does, I still want her to know that , there will and <u>should</u> be days that you are tired and you must stop and take care of yourself first! I will make sure that when she sees me as her mother that she sees me when I am strong, tenacious and fearless. But also that she sees me when I am tired and knows that it's okay to say I am tired, weak, fearful sometimes. She must see me put myself first so that I am physically and emotionally healthy for myself and for them.

We are what we learned, we are who we watched. We bring all of this with us to our adult life and relationships. Being aware of those influences, good and bad, are essential to becoming a whole, content peaceful

person no matter what roles you assume on the stage of life.

CHAPTER 2

Staying at Home With Them, Keeping in Touch with Me

- *A Full House*

I had just gotten out of the hospital after a C-section with my third child. My mother was here from California to help with the kids and household tasks. In the house we now have a six year old son, Tyler, Alexis an eighteen month old "very active" daughter, my ten year old niece Jordan who had joined our family five days earlier, and now our latest and "LAST" son Xavier who was four days old. 'What was I thinking ?

Fact:

In the six months of life, infants are fed at least 14,400 times.

- **A Quiet Walk Downstairs**

After being upstairs in our master bedroom for three days straight , looking at caramel brown walls and surviving the permanent smell of dirty diapers (*which has lingered around our house for almost two years now,*) I decided to venture downstairs to walk around and see what my mother and the other kids were doing. I walked down the stairs, holding a pillow around my stomach to help absorb some of the pain from my stapled incision, and protect myself from my curious eighteen-month year old. I sat down on the couch, so glad to be with my mom (an adult !) that I could talk to.

Before I could say a word, my six year old son and 18 month old daughter come rolling out into the foyer screaming and wrestling over a piece of paper. I just sat and looked at them flopping around the floor, made a quick assessment to see if anyone

14

was bleeding or wounded, looked at my Mom

helplessly and smiled to avoid crying…..at this

moment I knew life in my household had taken a

drastic turn toward chaos.

- **On Guard -Keeping Baby Safe**

When we brought Xavier home, Alexis kept

looking at him wondering what he was. When she

could get close she would nudge him to see what he

would do. When he would cry or move she would

jump back and smile in amazement. She has always

been very curious so she got bolder and bolder as

the days went on. We usually put the baby in the

infant carrier so that either my mother or I could be

on constant guard duty to protect him from his

persistent older sister. One day my mother was

cooking dinner and in my delirious state of lack of

sleep, I walked away from him in the carrier to go

to the bathroom. As soon as my daughter saw her opportunity she pounced and starting pulling Xavier out of the carrier. As I came out the bathroom, I heard my Mom, yell "Watch out!" All I saw was my infant son tilted in his carrier being pulled to the ground by Alexis. It all seemed like slow motion, I screamed "Stop Lexi !"as I hurdled over the side of the couch and loveseat to catch the carrier before it could hit the floor. Alexis was startled by my scream so she let go and he plopped back into his carrier and landed safely on the couch. Now you may ask, how did I hurdle the couches with 25 staples/stitches from a two week old c-section ? The answer is: I have no clue how I did it, but I did and didn't feel a thing. The kids looked at us like we were crazy. Xavier went back to sleep and Alexis ran off to find a toy to play with.

Fact:

The average pre-schooler requires his or her mother's attention every four minutes or 210 times a day. This is about fifty times as often as they will call Mom in a whole year after they've grown up and moved away.

- **My First Monday Morning**

      The first Monday morning after my mother returned to California, I woke up to Xavier crying for a bottle, Alexis calling 'Mommy" at the top of her lungs from her crib, and Tyler and Jordan needing to be pushed into gear in order to get dressed, eat breakfast, and catch the bus to school by 7:50am. I sat on the side of our bed thinking how lucky my husband was to be able to go to work and escape this madness for a couple of hours, and asking myself, 'How are you going to be able to do this on three hours of sleep? Am I crazy?

Fact:

The number of mothers staying at home has increased for the first time in 25 years. That means the number of sleep deprived women driving and wandering through the malls and supermarkets has also increased. Be afraid, be very afraid.

▪ **Where Do I Put the Baby?**

Now that my mother was gone, where do I put the baby so Alexis can't get to him? So it became quite a juggling act as to which one of them I could take downstairs first, then go back upstairs to get the other one. I use baby monitors so I can hear what the other one is doing while I am securing the area.

- **No Justice, No SLEEP!**

    When my mother was here and on weekends when my husband is home in the late night and early morning to help me, I am sometimes able to sleep during the day, napping when the baby naps. BUT during the week, when I wake up in the early morning, I can't go back to sleep until my husband gets home from work to help me. I wake up at 6 am to feed the Xavier after being up with him every two to three hours through the night. Shortly after at 6:30 am I have to wake up the older kids to get them ready for school. Then Alexis wakes up between 7:15 am and 7:30 am and wants her cup of milk and breakfast. She is well rested ready to play and watch Barney, Elmo and the Wiggles! I get her dressed and the phone starts ringing throughout the day, friends, family, telemarketers, etc... Well now

Xavier is sleeping soundly. I am up with Alexis trying to keep myself awake and alert and keep her occupied.

Once Alexis is ready for her nap around noon after lunch, it's now time for Xavier to wake up and eat again. I scarf some food down, caffeine, and move on to feeding him, changing diapers and giving him a cloth bath. I also have to make all necessary newborn doctor appointments for him, make sure Alexis appointments are made for her immunization shots. Jordan requires several doctor appointments and follow-ups due to a special medical condition. Tyler also has his regular dentist and doctor appointments. I have to pick up pharmacy medicine for everyone. Oh Yeah! and make doctor appointments for me, to remove staples and for the six-week post-partum check up etc.

By 2:30pm I am a walking zombie and time bomb! The older kids are home from school now and I have to weed through stacks of school flyers, notes, homework to see what school fundraiser, party, PTSA function is going on now and what I have to sign, what I won't sign etc. and by now Alexis is awake and ready to play again. By 4:00pm I am helping with homework assignments, giving Alexis her afternoon snack, and feeding Xavier again. Probably on my fortieth poo-poo or pee-pee diaper change of the day. Now I must find something quick and nutritious to cook for dinner. Every minute after 5:00 pm I am listening for my husband Carl to open the garage door and come in and rescue me or jump into the ocean of madness with me.

Sometimes I actually get a quick shower at around 6:30 pm when Carl gets home or sometimes it is as late as 10:00 pm. When my body decides that I can no longer stay awake I just crash for a few hours before I have to stay up with Xavier through the night feedings again.

Fact:

There are an estimated 6.8 million stay at home moms. That means that each of the 50 states has and average of 136,000 women who wander around singing "La la la la, la la la la, Elmo's World, Elmo's World".

- **Daddy's Home**

On Friday and Saturday nights and holidays, Carl is on guard all night for all the kids and I just veg out. This works for us but everyone has to come to their own agreement as a couple. This works for us because, we learned it doesn't make sense for both of us to be walking zombies at the same time.

When he gets home from work, I literally hand over everything, go to the bedroom and pass out. Unfortunately it definitely kills any chance for romance. Some days we are barely able to greet each other.

Now that Xavier is older and sleeps better, I insist that my husband have some time to unwind when he comes home. Even though he has never asked for it, I think it's important. We are gradually learning to block out time for us at night just to talk and stay in touch with one another "NO KIDS Allowed!"

We also agreed that even though he has to go to work the next morning, if I find that I can't wake up and feed the baby or take care of the kids in the middle of the night, he jumps right in and does it because, I also have to "work" the next morning it just so happens that I live at my job.

Fact:

Lillian walks an average of 15,000 steps a day. That is the equivalent of six miles. The Redding family does and average of fifteen loads of laundry per week.

Being a stay at home mom is one of the most difficult jobs in the world. This chart shows what it would cost to pay for the services provided by stay at home moms who work 80+ hours per week.

Job title	Annual salary
Child Day Care Worker	$20,259
Teacher	$44,824
Taxi Driver	$27,346
Facilities Manager	$73,239
Short-order Cook	$27,477
Laundry Attendant	$17,917
Janitor	$22,440
Counselor	$27,638
CEO	$545,268
Administrative Assistant III	$37,143
Accounting Clerk III	$34,842
Licensed Practical Nurse	$38,111
Plumber I	$33,155

Automotive Mechanic I	$30,725
Cake Decorator	$21,340

Jobs listed in order from largest to smallest component of a stay-at-home mom's job. All salaries are national averages. Source: Salary.com, 2004.

While the work is rewarding, it is also exhausting. You are constantly fulfilling needs of others. Feeding, changing, entertaining, disciplining, monitoring, loving, maintaining transporting in an endless cycle of giving.

While most women handle this in their own way, there are pitfalls to beware of. Places where you can lose perspective and lose yourself. We present these descriptions not as criticism but as troubleshooting guide. Do you see yourself here?

- The Hover Mother

    This mom is constantly one step behind their kids, fussing over clothes, toys, trying to protect from everything including life. Most first time mothers are very protective washing, rinsing, sterilizing everything in sight. They buy every new gadget, have every medication for every possible disease.

If you have several more children, the hover mechanism is usually disengaged. Dropped pacifiers are wiped off rather than boiled for 30 minutes. Sniffles and other ailments are expected and routinely dealt with when children play together.

But the Hover Mother continues to cover her children in maternal plastic wrap. She is the overzealous room mom who knows more than the teacher. The parent whose child is smarter and more special than all the others, thereby deserving more attention.

- The Martha Stewart Mother

The new icon of domestic perfection is Martha Stewart. She cooks, cleans, gardens, weaves her own Christmas wreaths and even makes her own candles.

Everything in her home is color coordinated, everything she serves is flawlessly presented. And she does it all by herself with a little help from a staff of several hundred professionals.

You recognize the Martha Stewart Mom by her tireless effort to keep her home looking like a magazine cover. Her house is a showplace, not a home. Often her family doesn't feel comfortable and is restricted to certain rooms or activities. She has a flag over her door for every season and holiday. She rushes to be the first one to have her outside Christmas decorations up.

She is in constant motion. There is always another pillow to plump, one more casserole to perfect. She searches for the centerpiece for every occasion and brags about where she bought her shoes and how much her draperies cost.

You might also find that her kids are in every activity. She rushes from soccer to baseball to ballet to karate. She never takes time to relax, to recharge and eventually she burns out.

- <u>The Busy Body</u>

She is the one whose call you don't answer; the one who rushes over to engage you when you walk to the mailbox; the one who is forever organizing and coordinating. She seems baffled when you don't want to be part of the block party or organize rotating play dates.

She is obsessed with what others are doing. She knows who built a fence, or got a new car or enlarged their deck. She constantly speculates on how others can afford to do all these things. She drops in unexpectedly and doesn't know when to leave. She calls often to borrow things so she can see what is in your home.

Eventually she is shunned and avoided.

- The Drama Mama

You never ask her how she is because she always has a story. There is always a health problem or some type of family drama. Her children are having trouble at school. Her husband is having problems at work. Her parents are getting older and more dependent on her.

She isn't happy unless she is miserable. There is no sunshine just gloom. No matter what your troubles, hers are greater, heavier and longer lasting. She engages you in long conversations about her issues. She might ask for advice but doesn't really want any.

It is common for her to be the leading expert on any subject from children's cold medication to choosing a nursing home. Nobody has more knowledge or trouble that she does. She loves an audience and will attend any gathering or meeting. She is seldom silent and will direct any conversation, no matter how unrelated, to be about her suffering.

If there is no problem to solve or crisis to resolve she feels useless. Her need to be needed overwhelms her ability to be content.

- Mother On Empty

30

Her eyes are tired. She is either overly cheerful or extremely quiet. She is easily distracted and shows little interest outside of everyday routine duties. She is often very sensitive or emotional. She may also be subject to mood swings. It is as though her post partum depression never leaves. She is constantly fighting against her own exhaustion and depression.

She is angry with her husband for not recognizing her plight. She resents her children for sucking up every ounce of her energy and demanding every moment of her time. She then feels guilty about feeling angry and resentful and so her depression deepens and she tries harder to suppress her feelings.

You might notice that she is distracted and lethargic. She may complain of aches and pains or have frequent colds and headaches. Her tank is empty and she is pushing her life uphill.

- <u>Mona Desmond Mom</u>

In the classic film Sunset Boulevard, Mona Desmond is a fading movie star who just can't face the reality that her career is over. She reminds everyone around her of past glories and achievements.

This is the mom who says "I may be just a stay-at- home Mom now but I used to be somebody." She constantly tells you about her achievements in the corporate world, her academic degrees or her athletic prowess before she became a mother.

She recites a list of credentials of past jobs, the degrees they earned, the people they knew all this to justify that they are worthy. They consider their stay-at-home status as a kind of martyrdom.

Let me say again, being a parent, especially a parent that stays home with children, is the hardest job in the world. But your job mustn't define you. You aren't just someone's mom or wife or partner. You are an individual with hopes, dreams, needs and rights.

Your kids, PTA, perfect house or past achievements can't fill up a hole in your soul. You must have a time and place to charge your batteries. You must make sure that those you care for don't take you for granted. You must exert your rights and needs as a pivotal member of your family. You need time for relaxation, decompression and doing things that bring you pleasure. You are not a machine.

You are not a bad mother if:

- Your children get on you last nerve and you need to be away from them. There are only so

many times you can hear "Mommy!" before you
need a break,

– Your kids are not in every possible activity
available. There are only so many hours in a
day. Carefully choose one or two activities that
both you and your children enjoy and schedule
comfortably. Consider this:

- Outside activities take time away
  from family time
- Some activities conflict with
  homework, sleep etc (8 pm baseball
  games on school nights)
- Some activities are expensive
- It takes considerable time and energy
  to pick up and drop off.

– You say no to what is popular. If you think a
book, movie or video game is not appropriate,
don't buy it. If you give in to peer pressure,

how will you teach your children not to do the same thing.

- You sometime get take out food . You aren't a machine. There are days when preparing a meal is just not an option. Being too tired or stressed or rushed to cook is not failure it's normal. Take out food has veggies too. Chinese, Thai, pizza, family style restaurants are all sources of healthy, tasty meals.

- You plan purchases and activities for your convenience. Choose a car because it works for you even if it isn't stylish or prestigious. Choose a house built for your ease. For example if the washer, dryer are in the basement, how many steps does that add to your day?

You have to put yourself first. Your family cannot drink from an empty well. You must be complete in mind, body and spirit to be of any use. You are teaching your sons and daughters about how women act and are to be treated.

One day children will be gone, what will you do with the rest of your life? Find out how to be content with where you are and who you are. If you aren't content, work at discovering the problem and have the courage to solve it.

Most of the time your mate doesn't get it. They have to be educated. They might say, "If I bring home the money and all you have to do is stay home what is the problem?" They may say, "I help as much as I can but I'm tired when I come home." Remind them that you work as hard as they do. Your contribution to the family is as important as theirs. You are also tired, stressed and drained. Negotiate with your partner so that you both remain whole and healthy.

Stand your ground on what you need. Buy a few hours of childcare every week so you can go grocery shopping in peace. Decide which night of the week you will turn over the kids to your mate and go out to a movie etc. by yourself. Take a class. Take a nap. Find a reliable babysitter or family member who will take the kids while the two of you go to dinner or a movie together.

In a truly committed relationship, raising children, caring for a home and making that home a happy, healthy place is a joint responsibility. Stand up, speak out, establish boundaries and take care of your health and your sanity.

CHAPTER 3

WAHMS (Work-At-Home-Moms)

It seems to be the perfect solution: a job that you can do from home. You can have the best of both worlds; stay home with your children and contribute financially to the family. On the internet are pages and pages of success stories about women who make huge sums of money every month working only a few hours per day.

But great caution must be used when considering this alternative. Here are six things to consider before committing to a work from home venture.

Examine Your Motives

Are up looking for a job to supplement the family income or are you looking for something to fulfill your need for intellectual, emotional or spiritual satisfaction? Are you looking for a business opportunity where you will build an organization to manage? Do you have an idea that you want to develop into a business? Honest answers to questions such as these are essential before you make an action plan.

Beware of scams

Most websites advertising work-from-home enterprises lead you through pages and pages of testimonials and verbiage that really don't give much information. At some point you will be asked for contact information or required to purchase a packet of information, often with a stated money back guarantee.

Read carefully before you commit. Be suspicious of a site that won't reveal any specifics about the product or service being offered. Giving you contact information might mean being bombarded with unwanted emails and phone calls. You can use a generic Yahoo, Hotmail etc address that can be checked online without downloading the email. Be suspicious if there is no phone number on the website or if the number you call takes you in circles.

Ask for references. Are there people in your area who are currently engaged in this activity? Do they have meetings or training classes? In which state is the company registered? Who are the officers? Know who you are going into business with.

Do the math

Once you have a clear idea of the nature of the business venture and a realistic estimate of the profit, ask yourself if the rewards are worth the effort. Can you do this business while taking care of the children? Will it require you to pay for daycare for even a few hours per week? How will it affect your income tax situation?

Assess the Effects

How will this new venture impact your daily work schedule? Adding another task will impact nap time, shopping time, meal time etc. Will it require a new sharing of household responsibilities? Will the new job become one more task added to an already crowded daily schedule?

Before committing to any new venture, all those effected must be included in the decision. Their willingness and ability to take on more responsibility, change their schedule and support your decision is essential.

Reassess At Three Months

After three months working from home do a thorough evaluation of your situation. Ask these questions:

- Is the financial gain worth the effort?
- How has the work affected me physically, mentally and spiritually?
- How has the work affected other members of my family?

<u>Safety First</u>

Some work at home jobs begin very innocently but lead down dark paths. Women have been lured into dangerous situations with promises of extra money or special training. Jobs involving secluded or deserted locations must be avoided. Any work involving sex based phone calls, arranged dating or other risky behavior are extremely dangerous no matter how lucrative.

These traps are particularly attractive if you are feeling overwhelmed or underappreciated. The purveyors of these schemes are experts at seduction, preying on need and vulnerability. Don't become a victim.

CHAPTER 4

Working Outside the Home

The purpose of this chapter is not to support or refute the claim that the disintegration of the American family is due to mothers working outside the home. Our purpose is to give guidance so that you can make an informed decision. The assessment process is similar to working from home model, but there are several additional matters to consider.

Do the Math

It isn't enough just to count the extra income from a job, you also have to count the additional expenditures involved. These expenses may include:

- Daycare for children (see Chapter 6)
- After school care for older children
- Double gasoline and vehicle maintenance
- Additional clothing expenses
- Additional income tax

If the amount you actually bring home doesn't significantly change your financial situation, reconsider your options.

Do the Daily Schedule

How will your family's day look when you are employed full time? Ask these questions. Write out a timetable and review it with your family.

- When do children have to be at daycare/school?
- What are the traffic patterns along the route to and from work and to and from school/daycare?
- When do adults have to be at work?
- When do children have to picked up from school or other activities?
- What are the penalties for a late pick-up?
- How much overtime will be required at work?
- How will meals be prepared/bought?

Map Out Plan B

With both parents working, there must be a contingency plan. Children get sick, have medical appointments, days off from school and school vacation.

The school vacation issue is complicated by many school districts with year-round school. "Vacation" for your child may come not in the summer when camps and churches have programs available, but in January, or March or September. What is your plan for these situations?

You often don't know a child is sick until they wake up in the morning. Or they become ill at school and must be picked up. Who's work schedule is flexible enough to take care of these situations? Further, if your child is in daycare, the rules are:

- A child sent home with a fever can return if their temperature has been normal for 24 hours
- A child sent home with oozing from the eye can return if there has been no oozing or redness for 48 hours
- A child sent home with vomiting or diarrhea can return if those symptoms are absent for 24 hours

It's not a matter of a few hours but often several days that alternative arrangements must be made. The situation becomes more complex if one or both of you have jobs that require travel. Children never get sick at a convenient time.

Does your job have the option of telecommuting? If so, can you choose the days to work from home or do you need prior approval? Is there someone who can substitute for you at critical meetings ?

These are difficult issues. They must be addressed and resolved before you commit to a job. If you wait to deal with them as they occur, it will often cause damaging complications in your professional and family life.

Again, this situation requires that you work out with the family, especially your spouse or partner, how household responsibilities will be reallocated. Shopping, cooking, child care, leisure time and housework have to be taken care of.

How will time on the weekend be divided?

Everyone needs time to decompress, relax and do things for fun. If you have young children who usually wake up early even on the weekends, those responsibilities must be equitably divided. Even during the week, adults must have time to change gears from work to home mode. Maybe it's only fifteen minutes to change

clothes, take a breather and refocus.

If you are both clear how things will be done from the beginning, there will be no surprises. Things change, adjustments will be made, compromise is the key. Talk, assess, agree, have a plan before you commit to a job.

It is crucial that as a couple you must find time to nurture your relationship. There must be time to talk, to share, to be intimate, even time to disagree and resolve issues. Use some of your resources to go out to dinner or a movie together. Make a date and, if possible, have lunch together during the week. After the children are in bed,

47

spend time together talking, necking or just sitting together in silence. In the rush of work and responsibility don't lose each other.

CHAPTER 5

Single Parents

There are many varieties of single parents. While each story is unique, there are basic similarities across the spectrum. This chapter deals with the reality of parenting alone not matter how you arrived at your present situation.

You can't be two people. No matter how hard you try you can't really be both mother and father. That doesn't mean that you can't be a good parent and raise healthy well-adjusted children. It does mean that if you spread yourself too thin, everyone loses.

Don't try to be Super Parent. Guilt often leads us to bring children gifts all the time, allow them to do whatever they want, acquiesce to all their demands. That kind of behavior won't make up for anything. It will produce maladjusted children and frustrated parents. You must be even more resolute in setting limits and sticking to them. There is usually no back-up. It's all on you.

If you do have another parent sharing custody, it is important that you agree on protocol and procedures. While this may not always be possible, every attempt should be made to see that your rules of behavior or discipline aren't completely undone during time spent with the other parent or a grandparent. If agreement can't be reached, it becomes even more important that you stand your ground at home.

As a single parent, how you explain what happened is up to you and depends on your situation. Widows, divorced persons, single parents by choice all have different stories. Some of the stories aren't easy to relate. Consultation with a counselor or mental health professional may be needed. But it is essential that your children know their limits and your expectations.

We all make mistakes. Marriages break up for many reasons. Relationship begin and end for many reasons. If you feel the need to apologize for past actions or behavior, do so. But don't let the past be used as a weapon against you in the present

Be very selective about who you introduce to your children. If the children have lost a parent through death or divorce, they are particularly vulnerable. A new person in your life might be seen as an unwanted replacement for a deceased parent or competition for a divorced parent. If this is the first date you don't know where the relationship is going, it is in everyone's best interest to proceed with caution and discretion.

Also, there is a safety issue, even for single dads. Predators of all types look for vulnerability. Letting people into your home gives them access to a large amount of personal information. Even casual conversation can reveal who lives in the home, their schedules and what security measures are in place.

A little paranoia can be a good thing. In the early stages of dating, meet at the restaurant or theatre rather than being picked up at home. Give the person a cell phone rather than a home phone number. Be careful how much information you share about your children and home situation. If you are a woman, either don't list your number in the phone book or only use your first initial so that gender isn't apparent.

Bringing someone home for the night or co-habitating is a very serious step indeed. There are many alternatives for intimate encounters than your own home. Whatever you do in front of your children, they will talk about, remember and probably imitate. You are teaching your daughters how to operate with men. You are teaching your sons how to treat women. You are teaching your children how to value and treat their bodies.

From a self-care perspective, there are sexually transmitted diseases that not only can't be cured but can kill. Insisting that partners use protection and/or taking blood tests if the relationship becomes serious isn't being over cautious. It is the only way that makes sense. Run from anyone who refuses to take precautions. If they are willing to risk their lives, they don't care about yours.

Single parents can become so overwhelmed that they begin to seek immediate relief for their problems without considering the long term effects. They begin to look for a partner just to help them get through the day; someone, anyone to share the burden. Such desperation can lead to very unhealthy situations. Financial or emotional dependence is not a firm foundation for a relationship. It gives one person a great deal of power and can easily lead to physical and psychological abuse.

A single parent must also consider that whomever you bring into your home will interact with your children. The degree of interaction ranges from being picked up/dropped off in a dating situation to co-habitation of whatever degree. Be very aware of the person's behavior towards your children. Is there too much interest in the children? Is there more attention given to children of one gender? Is there no interest in the children? What is the response when duties/activities for your children conflict with or take precedence over dating activities? What will be the consequences if your children become attached to someone and your relationship with that persons ends or changes?

This is very complicated. Being a single parent doesn't signal an end to your social life. You have a right and a need for social activity and fun. It is necessary if you are to be a whole, healthy person. But, like any parent, your behavior impacts your children.

Healthy lifestyles are about balance. This is especially key for single parents. The financial and parenting pressures push and pull from every direction. Any change in lifestyle must be carefully examined and all the ramifications evaluated.

For instance, before taking on a second job, consider what it will really involve. After deducting transportation, childcare costs etc. will you bring home enough additional money to make a difference? How much more time will you spend away from your family? Will you create a situation where your children are left alone or with less than adequate supervision? How will working the extra hours affect your physical and emotional health?

The key is to do the best you can with what you have. There are no Super Parents. Certainly some parents do a better job than others parents but no parent is perfect. Don't try to be the first. You have a tough job and it is more important than ever that you take care of yourself.

CHAPTER 6

Child Care

Throughout the proceeding chapters, the issue of childcare has been mentioned many times. USA Today reports that nearly 12 million children under age five are in some type of regular childcare each week.

The quality and cost of childcare varies greatly according to where the family lives. The National Associate of Child Care Resource and Referral Agencies reports that child care fees for one infant range from $3,803 to $13,480 per year. Average fees for an infant are higher that the average among families spend on food each year.

The following table shows the state –to-state cost of child care for a four year old:

State-to-state costs vary

Ranking of cost of child care for a 4-year-old: (1 = highest; 50 = lowest)

State	Average annual cost of preschool care	%. of median single parent family income spent on preschool care	%. of median two-parent family income spent on preschool care	Ranking of preschool care as a percentage of income
Alabama	$3,016	18.30%	4.80%	50
Alaska	$6,684	23.00%	8.40%	22 (tie)
Arizona	$5,876	26.20%	9.40%	12 (tie)
Arkansas	$3,384	22.30%	6.10%	48
California	$7,576	31.10%	10.90%	3
Colorado	$7,020	27.70%	9.20%	15 (tie)
Connecticut	$8,459	29.90%	9.00%	19
Delaware	$5,515	23.80%	7.00%	40 (tie)
Florida	$4,948	21.60%	7.80%	32
Georgia	$4,025	20.30%	6.20%	45 (tie)
Hawaii	$5,620	22.60%	7.30%	36
Idaho	$4,803	28.20%	8.40%	22 (tie)
Illinois	$6,806	31.60%	9.20%	15 (tie)
Indiana	$5,408	25.60%	8.40%	22 (tie)
Iowa	$5,375	25.70%	8.40%	22 (tie)
Kansas	$4,446	18.30%	6.90%	43
Kentucky	$4,710	32.40%	8.10%	28
Louisiana	$4,760	30.30%	7.70%	33 (tie)
Maine	$6,344	34.80%	9.40%	12 (tie)
Maryland	$6,515	20.20%	7.20%	37 (tie)
Massachusetts	$9,628	40.70%	10.60%	4
Michigan	$6,216	29.10%	8.70%	20
Minnesota	$8,832	31.10%	11.40%	2
Mississippi	$3,904	26.70%	6.80%	44
Missouri	$3,967	18.70%	6.10%	47
Montana	$4,486	26.20%	8.00%	29 (tie)
Nebraska	$5,100	26.20%	7.90%	31
Nevada	$3,200	14.30%	5.30%	49
New Hampshire	$7,014	24.90%	8.50%	21
New Jersey	$8,985	32.80%	9.60%	8 (tie)
New Mexico	$5,054	35.10%	9.10%	17 (tie)

57

New York	$8,530	40.40%	11.50%	1
North Carolina	$5,876	31.80%	9.40%	12 (tie)
North Dakota	$4,784	26.30%	7.60%	35
Ohio	$6,159	31.10%	9.10%	17 (tie)
Oklahoma	$4,073	23.50%	7.00%	40 (tie)
Oregon	$5,160	26.00%	8.20%	27
Pennsylvania	$6,800	31.40%	9.60%	8 (tie)
Rhode Island	$7,800	45.30%	10.30%	5 (tie)
South Carolina	$4,180	22.80%	6.20%	45 (tie)
South Dakota	$4,804	24.90%	7.70%	33 (tie)
Tennessee	$4,188	22.30%	7.00%	40 (tie)
Texas	$4,427	21.70%	7.20%	37 (tie)
Utah	$4,764	21.50%	8.00%	29 (tie)
Vermont	$6,537	27.70%	9.50%	10 (tie)
Virginia	$7,852	34.60%	10.30%	5 (tie)
Washington	$6,891	32.70%	9.50%	10 (tie)
West Virginia	$3,886	26.70%	7.10%	39
Wisconsin	$6,968	31.00%	9.80%	7
Wyoming	$5,438	29.80%	8.40%	22 (tie)

Note: Costs of child care are based on the price of care in a licensed child care center. The information was provided by the State CCR&R Network, except where noted, in early 2005; 1 cost of preschool care is based on information provided by local CCR&R agencies in 2005; 2 cost of infant and preschool care is based on information provided by local CCR&R agencies in 2005. Source: National Association of Child Care Resource and Referral Agencies

These costs are averages. The quality and cost of care varies greatly. This is further complicated by logistics. The most inexpensive child care may not be conveniently located. Parents have to consider traffic patterns, proximity to work routes etc. If there are older children in school and/or after school programs, the timing for pick-up and drop off is critical.

How do you choose a child care provider? Here are a few tips but this list is by no means exhaustive:

- Do the math – What can you realistically afford to pay?

- Visit the facility unannounced. Ask for a tour and take notes. Look for cleanliness, classroom equipment, quality of food and notice how the facility smells.

- When you have a short list, check with the state regulatory agencies for any reports of violations.

- Be sure you understand the rules of the facility regarding children who are ill. Most centers require a child to be free of fever for 24 hours and free of vomiting/diarrhea for 48 hours before they can return to school.

- Have a plan for holidays and days when the kids are too sick for day care. Ask family members and price paid babysitters.

- For short term solutions, check with local churches for special drop-off programs or Mom's Afternoon Out options.

- Couples Night Out is offered by some churches/community organizations. It provides child care services for a few hours in the evening so parents can have time to themselves.

- Look for companies and placement agencies with flexible work hours or that offer day care. You can take a more proactive stance and research companies who have in house day care and flex hours, find out how they started and present a proposal to your employer.

Choose child care with great care. Check your children for cleanliness and general health regularly. If they can talk, ask them what happens at school. If you hear anything that concerns you, make inquiries. If possible, make spot checks by arriving at unexpected times or a meal times or during nap time. This is recommended even if things are going well.

Listen and look for signals from your children. If a child still cries when being dropped off or doesn't want to go to school even after a suitable adjustment time, be very concerned. Better to be called an overprotective parent than to put your children in harms way.

CHAPTER 7

SINK AND DINK

There are several new life styles that have emerged from the shadows into the light of respectability. Two of these are SINK and DINK: Single Income No Kids and Double Income No Kids.

At one time it was considered almost heretical. It certainly was seen as selfish and reflective of serious character defects. How could anyone, especially a woman choose not to have children ? Being a mother was considered the ultimate and only true fulfillment for a woman. Having a family was what all responsible men worked for and wanted.

Things have changed. Deciding not to be a parent is now a legitimate and respected choice for men and women. It is not an alternative reserved for those who didn't find a suitable mate or were infertile. It is indeed a choice for those who find that a commitment to parenting isn't one they are willing to make. It doesn't mean they don't like children or are disparaging of those who have kids. It most likely means that after an honest assessment, they have found that they aren't suited for raising children.

Not everyone is born with the parenting gene. It is possible to find fulfillment in a different way. Maybe through your career or service to others or dedication to achieving a specific goal that requires all of your effort or perhaps a combination of reasons.

This is a valid choice. There are so many who drift into childbearing and then regret the decision. There are so many children born to parents who aren't willing or able to care for them and become neglected and/or abused in so many ways.

Abuse is not just about beatings or molestation it can be about emotional neglect and humiliation. Abuse can happen in the wealthiest of homes when money and things replace time, love and discipline. Having a child is a lifetime commitment. It doesn't end at age eighteen or when they get a job and their own apartment.

Infertility is an increasingly common problem. We are bombarded with stories of people going to extraordinary lengths to have a child. While the scientific technology is available and adoption is always and option, the legal, moral and ethical implications are complex and often heartbreaking. Birth parents and surrogates who change their minds, sperm and egg donors who at some point want to find their offspring. There are those who find it might have been better to find other outlets for their parental energies.

Not being a parent either by choice or design does not relegate you to an empty, meaningless life. In 1940's Hollywood people who chose to stay single were portrayed either as self-sacrificing martyrs devoting themselves to good works or hard-hearted tyrants obsessed with wealth and power. That image is not only outdated but insulting.

The choice is yours and should be made without shame or

guilt.

CHAPTER 8

Sandwich Generation

The transfer of authority and transformation of roles between me and my mother occurred gradually and painfully. First came the death of my husband in 1978 followed two years later by the death of her husband, my father. We were raising my two children with little money and living in my mother's house. Several years later we moved to California where she was living in my house. Finally she suffered a seizure on Christmas Day 1993 and had to go to a nursing home.

I was her only child and she was of a generation steeped in the tradition of children taking care of their parents. Sometimes I wonder if the biological clock that pushed her to marry at thirty nine and have me at forty two was not just procreative but geriatric.

After I put her in the home, her campaign to make me feel guilty was relentless. In her mind, she belonged in the empty bedroom in my home. She wouldn't be any trouble and surely I could get some older lady in the neighborhood to come by and look in on her during the day.

The dichotomy is that the driving, sometimes mean-spirited stubbornness that I found so frustrating and hurtful to deal with is what has kept her alive and functioning all these years. I had to tame that tenacity for survival and not destroy her will to live. This woman who taught me how to be a daughter, a woman, a mother, a wife was facing the end of her life.

Often during this transition she hardened my heart, pushed me away while trying to smother me, until our roles had completed their reversal. I became the impatient parent and she the intractable child.

I remember the first time, she didn't recognize me. How many times had I wished she would stop calling me, claiming my time, vying for my complete attention. But when she looked at me with vacant, puzzled eyes and said "Tell me who you are?", I felt a overwhelming sense of loss.

I answered her question and received a brief smile of recognition and squeeze of the hand. But ten minutes later she said "I'd really like to know who you are?"

It was difficult to see what she had become. The independent spirit now confused and frustrated. The take charge manner now only a complaining, petulant echo. The ever vigilant eyes and ears dimmed and silenced by age and the slow growing, inoperable tumor in her brain.

I remember the busy, stylish woman bustling around the kitchen in the Chicago apartment where I grew up. Taking care of me and my father and her parents and my father's father and her brothers and sisters. Always having an opinion and expressing it forcefully, oblivious to how it would be received.

My childhood was filled with hours of listening to her relate stories of struggle, and discrimination in her native Alabama. She taught in rural schools in the 20's when the education of black children was of very low priority and all she had was a box of chalk, and blackboard eraser, a roll book and tattered hand-me-down books from the white schools. One of the few times I ever saw her cry was as she watched the culmination of the march from Selma to Montgomery, Alabama. As the throngs of people marched up Dexter Avenue demanding freedom for all, she remembered herself as a young girl being called names and forced to step off the sidewalk into the street.

Occasionally the old spark ignited again. "Oil my hair to the scalp." or "I need to come to your house this weekend to get away from all these crazy people here." And for a fraction of a second I was twelve again and my learned response to obey took over. But I was not twelve, I was fifty. And while she was still my mother, and ninety three years old, it is she who had to obey me.

She never complained about the frequency of my visits because time had lost its meaning. She would stare at the photographs of her grandchildren and great grandchildren and only fleetingly remember them.

I watched and endured and comforted, knowing that while I prayed for her passing to be swift and painless, it would leave a void in my existence that could never be filled. And would push me a little closer to the head of the line.

There have always been caregivers but the magnitude and complexity of caregiving has exploded in the last twenty years. Let's be clear who caregivers are. The following definitions and statistics are based on information from the Family Caregiver Alliance (www.caregiver.org) and should be considered estimates:

The term *caregiver* refers to anyone who provides assistance to someone else who is, in some degree, incapacitated and needs help: a husband who has suffered a stroke; a wife with Parkinson's disease; a mother-in-law with cancer; a grandfather with Alzheimer's disease; a son with traumatic brain injury from a car accident; a child with muscular dystrophy; a friend with AIDS.

Informal caregiver and *family caregiver* are terms that refer to unpaid individuals such as family members, friends and neighbors who provide care. These individuals can be primary or secondary caregivers, full time or part time, and can live with the person being cared for or live separately. *Formal caregivers* are volunteers or paid care providers associated with a service system.

The magnitude of caregiving is shown below:

- **52 million** informal and family caregivers provide care to someone aged **20+** who is ill or disabled.

71

- **29.2 million** family caregivers provide personal assistance to adults (**aged 18+**) with a disability or chronic illness.

- **34 million** adults (16% of population) provide care to adults **50+ years**.

- **8.9 million** caregivers (20% of adult caregivers) care for someone **50+ years who have dementia**.

- **5.8 - 7 million** people (family, friends and neighbors) provide care to persons **65+** who need assistance with everyday activities.

- Unpaid family caregivers will likely continue to be the largest source of long-term care services in the U.S. and are estimated to reach 37 million caregivers by 2050, an increase of 85% from 2000.

Women provide the majority of informal caregiving as these numbers indicate:

- More women than men are caregivers. An estimated 59% to 75% of caregivers are female.

- Research suggests that the numbers of male caregivers may be increasing and will continue to do so due to a variety of social demographic factors. One report documents a 50% increase in men becoming primary caregivers between 1984 and 1994.

- While men may be sharing in caregiving tasks more than in the past, women still shoulder the major burden of care. For example, while some studies show a relatively equitable distribution of caregiving between men and women, female caregivers spend 50% more time providing care than male caregivers. However, among caregivers 75+, both sexes provide equal amounts of care.

- Other studies have found that women caregivers handle the most difficult caregiving tasks (i.e., bathing, toileting and dressing) when compared with their male counterparts who are more likely to help with finances, arrange care, and other less burdensome tasks.

- A number of studies have found that female caregivers are more likely than males to suffer from anxiety, depression, and other symptoms associated with emotional stress due to caregiving.

With 10,000 Baby Boomers turning 50 every day and improved health care extending life, the age of caregivers is also an important consideration:

- While caregivers can be found across the age span, the majority of caregivers are middle-aged (35-64 years old).
- The average age of family caregivers caring for someone aged 20+ has been estimated at 43.
- Of those caring for someone aged 50+, the average age of family caregivers is estimated at 47.
- Many caregivers of older people are themselves elderly. Of those caring for someone aged 65+, the average age of caregivers is 63 years with one third of these caregivers in fair to poor health.

Being a caregiver is a difficult, demanding job. It is especially difficult if you also have other demands on your life. You have elderly parents who need you but your children are still at home. In addition you may have a job and a significant other who also needs your attention.

The choices become agonizing. Do you go to your son's basketball game or your mother's physical therapy session ? Do you move your elderly parent into your home or try to keep them in their own home? How do you handle siblings or other family members who don't help but criticize your choices?

One of the most agonizing choices to be made by caregivers is when to consider assisted living or a nursing home. There are situations where this is the only viable and reasonable action to take. We read the horror stories of neglect and abuse and the unbelievable cost of care but circumstances may dictate that a skilled nursing facility is the only way.

Those circumstances vary. It could be that no one is available during the day to care for the patient. Maybe the patient is suffering from dementia but is ambulatory and wanders away or injuries themselves trying to cook etc. Maybe your home simply doesn't have the space for a hospital bed or other equipment. Maybe the patient needs skilled care that no family member is qualified to administer. Maybe the patient is a person that for whatever reason is not welcome in your home. There are many things to consider.

If you are thinking of a nursing home, here are few basic tips to consider before making a final choice:

- Make sure that the insurance/Medicare etc is accepted by the facility and what the conditions of admission are. Some situations require that the patient not own property or have any resources in their name.

- Take a tour not only with your eyes but with your ears and nose. Listen to how the staff talks to the residents. Notice how the facility smells. Go to the food preparation area. Notice if the residents are involved in activities or just left to sit alone and unattended.

- Make unexpected visits around meal time, early in the morning or late in the evening. See if things are different from the scheduled tour.

- Ask for references. Talk to those who have placed relatives in the facility.

- Consider the location. How convenient will it be to visit from your job or home? Can someone reach the facility quickly in the event of an emergency?

- Make sure all powers of attorney, do not resuscitate orders, living wills etc are valid and known to the doctors at the facility.

- Realize that sometimes a nursing home is the best choice of everyone involved and should be considered without guilt or remorse.

Your health and well being is as important as that of the person you take care of , maybe more important. You are involved in a very complicated situation with many people. You must interact not only with the person you take care of but also with family members, insurance companies, health professionals and maybe lawyers or social workers. They all are an integral part of the life and care of the patient. But the most important person in this scenario is not the person who is ill; the most important person is you, the caregiver.

Try and imagine what would happen if you were not in this picture. Who would take your place? Who would provide the services that you do? What effect would such a change have? So you owe it to yourself and to the person you care for to make sure you are at your best.

Sometimes we spend so much time doing for others that we fail to do for ourselves. Especially caregivers put their needs aside in order to provide for others. Caregivers often feel guilty if they take time for themselves or indulge their own wants and needs.

Finally, here are two very important points to remember as a caregiver. First, know that you are not on the caretaker road alone. There are many support groups and agencies that you can go to for help. Talk to others in your situation. Vent your feelings. Learn from those who have been through what you have yet to face.

Secondly, there are times when choices must be based solely on what is best for you. While you want to do all you can to honor the wishes of the patient and the desires of other family members, if you are the primary caregiver the final choice is yours. You can never please everyone. You have to make those choices that create the most favorable situation for you to provide effective, efficient and timely care to the patient.

CHAPTER 9

Redefining Self

From childhood we are taught not to be selfish. You have to share your toys, break your cookie in half and let your little sister watch her favorite program. Doing things to help others with no desire for payment or reward makes you a better person. All of these things are good and true. We don't want a world of people whose only focus is what is good for them with no regard for the rights or feelings of others. But it seems that women especially have taken this behavior too literally. This commitment to self sacrifice and service is too often carried to such an extreme that women forget to be good to themselves. How do you know if you have gone to far? What are the signs of self neglect? It starts with writing yourself a reality check:

- <u>No one's life is perfect</u>

    The biggest movie star, the greatest athlete, the most influential national or religious leader all have problems. Look at the divorce rate among the rich and famous. Anyone, famous or not, who is successful in life is well grounded in reality. Life is not a sitcom or an infomercial.

No matter what Rachel Ray says , making a full meal in 30 minutes that doesn't involve a microwave is not always possible. Martha Stewart can take the vines from last spring and make a Christmas wreath but most of us just go buy one.

Men, you won't maintain six pack abs without a great deal of work for many years. You hair will lose its wave and possibly disappear. Bob Villa has thousands of dollars worth of tools and years of experience so don't expect to build a fence or a doll house with his precision.

Your children won't always be well behaved. Your house won't be absolutely clean and straight all the time. Your wardrobe won't be perfectly color coordinated and there will be days when even combing your hair will be an effort.

This doesn't mean you are a failure. It means you are human. There are only so many days in a year and so many hours in a day. Each one of us has to make a realistic assessment of what we can do mentally, physically, emotionally and spiritually. We have to strip away false and unreachable standards that others have of us or that we have set for ourselves and learn a new definition of self.

How we define self determines how we evaluate words like selfish or selfness or selfdom or self interest or self centered. It determines how we choose and prioritize. It determines where we place ourselves in relation to others. It profoundly influences our lives as children, siblings, parents, workers and participants in relationships.

- **<u>SELF - one's own interest, welfare or advantage</u>**

Your interests are things that are important to you. Do you regularly do things that are important to you, even small things? For instance, how many times have your bought the bread or ice cream or cereal that your kids or husband wants instead of what you want? How many times have you compromised just to keep peace even when you knew it wasn't to your benefit?

Your welfare is that which impacts your mental, physical, spiritual and emotional health. Being exhausted, depressed or in physical or emotional pain isn't normal or acceptable. How effective are you in looking after the welfare of others when you don't look after your own?

If something improves your situation, then it is to your advantage. To improve your situation is a good thing. It doesn't mean that you're taking something away from or harming someone else. It means making a positive choice that makes changes your life for the better.

In order to live your best life you must be fulfilled, content and healthy in order to be available to others in your life. Here is a four step plan to begin that process.

- **Stop, Evaluate Learn, , Follow through**

STOP

Take some time by yourself and consider your life. Ask yourself these questions and answer them honestly:

1. Am I doing what is important to me and for me? Am I doing those things that bring me joy?

2. What is the state of my health? When did I have my last complete physical? Am I depressed, sad, unfulfilled,

restless, sleepless? Am I hearing voices or hallucinating?

3. Is a change needed in my life? Where am I going and what do I hope to find there? You can make a journal of your thoughts and then go back and read what you wrote. What does your journal say about you and the life you lead?

EVALUATE

Once you have answered those critical questions, you have to take the information you have and gauge its accuracy and importance. What issues are you most impassioned about? Which circumstances require your immediate attention? Which things are going well in your life?

This is a time for brutal honesty. You may need to consult with a trusted friend or even a mental health or life

coaching professional. Where are you on

the road of your life? Are you headed in the

direction that is right for you or are you on

the wrong path ?

LEARN

To learn is to add to one's

knowledge or information. To learn is to

ascertain or verify facts by inquiry or

analysis. To learn is to detect or to become

aware of something that has been obscure,

secret or concealed.

At this point, you add meat to the

bare bones of your evaluation. If change is

needed how can it be accomplished? Are

there a series of steps to be taken? Who

should you talk to? What are the risks?

It is helpful at this stage to contact someone who has successfully accomplished what you want to do. Ask them questions and take copious notes. The internet is a wonderful source of information. If you don't have your own computer, go to the public library. You can get a free email account at yahoo or hotmail or many other sites. Remember that all information on line isn't accurate so be discerning. Check and double check with reputable websites. Send emails, make phone calls. Do your homework with diligence and care.

FOLLOW THROUGH

George Bernard Shaw said "People are always blaming their circumstances for what they are. I don't believe in circumstances. The people who get on in this world are the

87

people who get up and look for the circumstances they want, and, if they can't find them, they make them." Hold yourself accountable. Nothing will change if you don't proactively make a change.

No one will know what you need if you don't speak up. Old patterns of behavior will continue until you change them. People will continue to treat you the same way until you teach them to treat you differently. Make a plan, stick to it, revise it when necessary. Things didn't get the way they are overnight and they won't change overnight. Persist, push on, stand up for yourself, establish your boundaries and enforce them. If you don't who will?

Here are Ten Basic Rules for Self-Care:

I. Thou shall not be perfect, or even try to be

You are not superhuman. You can only do what you can do. You have a right to feel tired, overwhelmed, exhausted and irritated. You have a responsibility to rest, recuperate and revitalize. Take a drive. Take nap. Enjoy a cup of your favorite coffee at your leisure. The only perfect people are in commercials or Lifetime television movies. Allow yourself to be human.

II. Thou shall not try to be all things to all people

Daily prioritizing is essential. Everyone's needs and demands must be weighed against what is practical and doable. There will be days when work comes first, other days when children are the priority, days when your relationship with your mate takes priority. Most of all you must take time for you. Be good to yourself so you can be of some good to others.

III.   Thou shall sometimes leave things undone

It has been scientifically proven that dust will keep indefinitely if you don't get it wet. Housework, Christmas shopping, cooking dinner sometimes won't get done. The world will continue to turn. The sun will rise, the moon will shine and life as we know it on planet earth will proceed on schedule. If someone is upset because a task isn't completed, tell them to do it themselves. No matter how fast you run, there are still only 24 hours in a day.

IV. Thou shall insist on help from others

Taking care of a family is a group activity. One person doing everything is sure to result in burnout. Ask for help. While family members are not always cooperative, children and mates should be responsible for specific chores. Cleaning, car and yard maintenance even meal preparation are everyone's responsibility.

Young children can set the table, load or unload the dishwasher. Your mate can have designated days to either cook or bring home dinner. Teens can earn/maintain driving privileges by reminding you when servings is needed or checking car fluid levels weekly.

You can't do it alone so don't even try.

V. Thou shall learn to say "No."

Only you can gauge your energy level. Only you know when you have reached the end of your rope, tied a knot and are just hanging on. You can't continue to add on to your activities and responsibilities.

You have to learn to say NO and mean it. Arranging the rummage sale at church, organizing the Halloween potluck at work, baking cookies for the scout troop or having the entire family over for Thanksgiving just may not be possible. Those who love you will understand. Those who don't understand aren't worth your effort or attention.

VI. Thou shall switch thyself off, and do nothing regularly.

You must find your OFF button and use it regularly. Make time to sit down and do nothing. Doing nothing is not folding clothes while you watch TV. Doing nothing is not listening to music while you clean the house. Doing nothing is sitting with your feet up watching your favorite DVD or reading a great book. Doing nothing is taking a nap or a long bubble bath. Doing nothing, is doing something that gives you pure joy and pleasure.

Even appliances shut themselves off at times. If your refrigerator runs all the time, you'd call the repair person and pay the bill or buy a replacement. If you are run all the time and blow a fuse, repairs and replacements are not so easily made.

VII. Thou shall not even feel guilty for doing nothing, or saying no.

It is a weapon used for many years by parents, children and other master manipulators; guilt. One definition of guilt is an awareness of having done wrong or committed a crime, accompanied by feelings of shame and regret. The key here is that you may not really have done anything wrong but are just made to feel that you did.

Saying no or being unavailable will often inconvenience others and they will lash out at you for being selfish or playing the martyr. Develop alligator skin and let the harsh words bounce off. This is a skill that comes with time and practice but like anything else, it get easier the more you do it. Taking care of yourself is nothing to feel guilty about. It is something of which to be proud.

VIII. Thou shall schedule time for thyself and for thy support network.

No one understands your situation unless they have walked in your shoes. Support groups of all kinds can be located through the internet, the local hospital, the senior citizen' center or wellness center. Find a group and attend regularly. Even if you are handling your duties adequately and taking care of yourself, you can give strength to others while drawing encouragement from their experiences. This is especially important if you are a caregiver for someone with a chronic or disabling illness or injury.

There are groups that specialize in those caring for Alzheimer's patients, or children, or even caring for parents or adults who were abusive. There are many difficult choices and situations in life. Having a caring community to help you through those agonizing times is priceless.

IX. Thou shall be boring, untidy, inelegant, and unattractive at times.

Sometimes just getting from sunrise to sunset with your sanity intact is all that you can do. Make-up, hair dos and color coordinated wardrobes are just not priorities. We should all have those outfits that are made for comfort.

There are days when worn sweat pants, faded flannel shirts, fuzzy slippers and bulky socks are as comforting as macaroni and cheese or chocolate éclairs.

There are days when your primary purpose when you get up in the morning is to live until you can go to bed again and fall into blessed unconsciousness.

You won't be bubbly, outgoing, optimistic, stylish or inspiring on those days, but it you make it through without committing a felony or running away to Tahiti, it will be a victory. Allow yourself to be a grumpy, grouchy slightly offensive human being at times. There are times when you may have it all together but you forgot where you put it. Relax, it happens to the best of us.

X. Especially, thou shall not be thine own worst enemy. But, be thine own best friend.

You are your best advocate. Others won't know what you need or how you're feeling if you don't speak up. Make you your first priority as a caregiver. What do you need to accomplish your tasks? Trust your instincts. Ask for advice. Include your immediate family in your decision making process. Love yourself, embrace yourself, know your importance and demand that others respect you needs

and boundaries.

Women, we must be our own best friends, we have

to support each other's choices even when we disagree.

When a man decides to become a stay at home Dad he is

applauded for his courage but women who stay at home are

drawn into debates with other women who work outside the

home about who is the better parent. Do what works for

you. Poet and essayist e.e. cummings wrote "To be nobody

but yourself in a world which is doing its best day and night

to make you everybody else, means to fight the hardest

battle which any human being can fight and never stop

fighting." Be true to you.

We have to be our loudest advocate. What are the

laws in your state on stalking, domestic violence,

restraining orders, child support etc. ? How are childcare

facilities licensed and inspected? What can we do about

how women are portrayed in advertisements ?

We have to learn to say no and mean it. We have to learn to say "After me, you come first" and not feel guilty. We are teaching young girls how to be women. We are teaching young boys how to treat women. We will shape the future of the world.

Take care of yourself so you can be the best you can be for others. A very wise person said " The name of the game is taking care of yourself, because you're going to live long enough to wish you had." What is the point of living longer if the quality of life doesn't improve? Happiness is self made. You can create the life you want and deserve. People often say that people haven't found themselves. We submit that self is not found it is something each person creates for themselves. Take care of yourself.

RESOURCE LIST

National Family Caregivers Association
10400 Connecticut Avenue, Suite 500
Kensington, MD 20895-3944
Toll Free: 1-800-896-3650
Phone: 301-942-6430
Fax: 301-942-2302
General E-mail: info@thefamilycaregiver.org

Working Mother Media Inc.
60 East 42nd Street
27th Floor
New York, NY 10165
212.351.6400   www.workingmother.com

Child Care Aware
3101 Wilson Blvd. Suite 350
Arlington, VA 22201 www.childcareaware.org
1-800-424-2246; TTY: 1-866-278-9428
Assists parents in finding the best information on locating
quality child care and child care resources in their
community.

Single Parents Association (SPA)
4727 E. Bell Road, Suite 45, PMB 209
Phoenix, Arizona 85032
(623) 581-7445
Was formed to provide education, resources, friendship and
camaraderie, as well as, FUN activities for single parents
and their children

National Association of Child Care Resource and Referral
Agencies (NACCRRA)
NACCRRA
3101 Wilson Boulevard Suite 350
Arlington, VA 22201 -
(703-341-4100)
A network of over 800 Child Care Resource and Referral
agencies offering training , resources and standards of best
practices to those agencies in support of quality,
accountable services. In addition, NACCRRA promotes
national policies and partnerships facilitating universal
access to quality child care.

American Psychiatric Association
1000 Wilson Boulevard
Suite 1825
Arlington, VA 22209
Call Toll-Free: 1-888-35-PSYCH
From outside the U.S. and Canada call: 1-703-907-7300
Email: apa@psych.org   www.healthyminds.org

Childbirth Connection
281 Park Avenue South, 5th Floor
New York, NY 10010
p: 212.777.5000
f: 212.777.9320
www.childbirthconnection.org
A source for trustworthy up-to-date evidence-based
information and resources on planning for pregnancy,
pregnancy, labor and birth, and the postpartum period.
Founded in 1918, Childbirth Connection is a national not-
for-profit organization dedicated to improving maternity
care quality and value

The Alzheimer's Association
225 N. Michigan Ave., Fl. 17
Chicago, IL 60601-7633
tel: 312.335.8700
tdd: 312.335.5886
fax: 1.866.699.1246
www.alz.org
This is the leading voluntary health organization in
Alzheimer care, support and research.

*ElderCare*link
190 Front Street
Suite 201
Ashland, MA 01721
contactus@ElderCarelink.com
An internet-based referral service—free to consumers—
that specializes in eldercare case matching for elders and
their families. *ElderCare*link assists families in finding a
multitude of services, including assisted living, nursing
homes, adult day care, private duty nursing, care
management and homecare.

The Postpartum Stress Center
1062 Lancaster Avenue
Rosemont Plaza, Suite 2
Rosemont, PA 19010
Ph: 610.525.7527
Providing support, counseling and education to women
and their families who experience difficulties related to
pregnancy, pregnancy loss and the postpartum period.